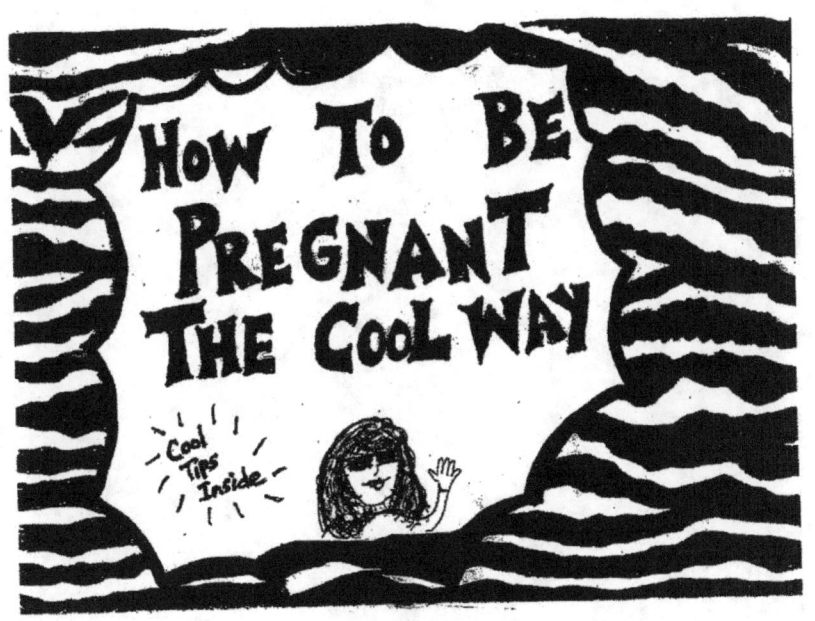

# By Dawnie C

This book is dedicated to
my family. They are my world!


2017

I've been cool most of my life.

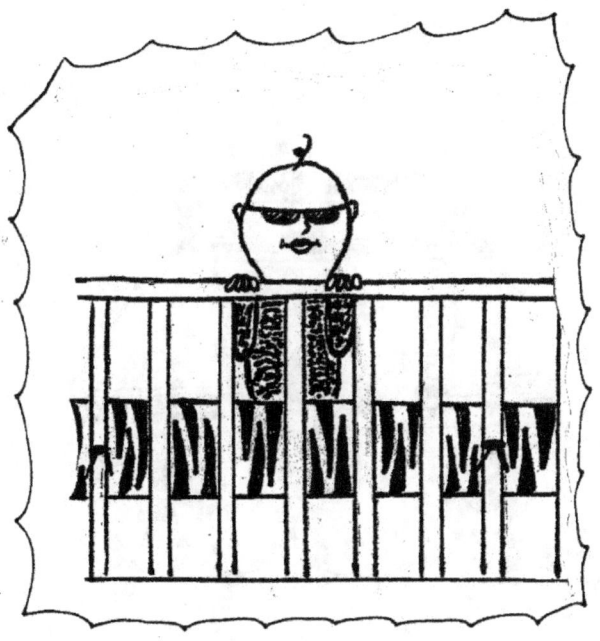

I drive a cool car.

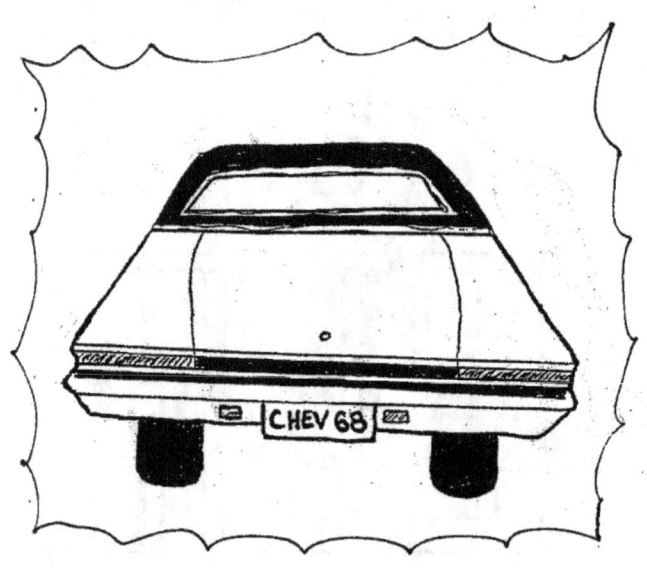

My whole family is cool.

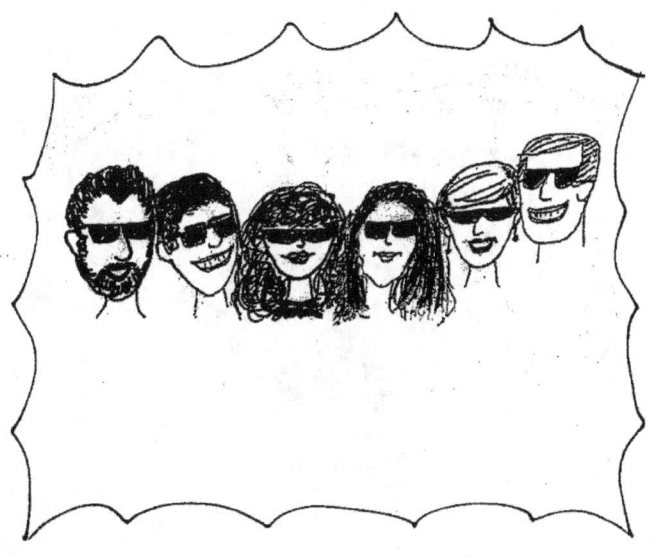

But the tricky thing for me
was being cool while I was
pregnant. Pregnancy does
its best to keep you uncool.
You can't wear high heels,
you can't color your hair,
you gain weight and
sometimes you even throw
up! Forget about that
morning cup of coffee!
It's decaf for the next nine
months. Confidence is the
key to being cool. Here are
some other tips to help
you be pregnant the cool way!

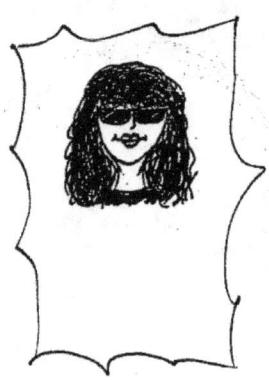

One day, when I was
shopping with my mom,
I became ill.

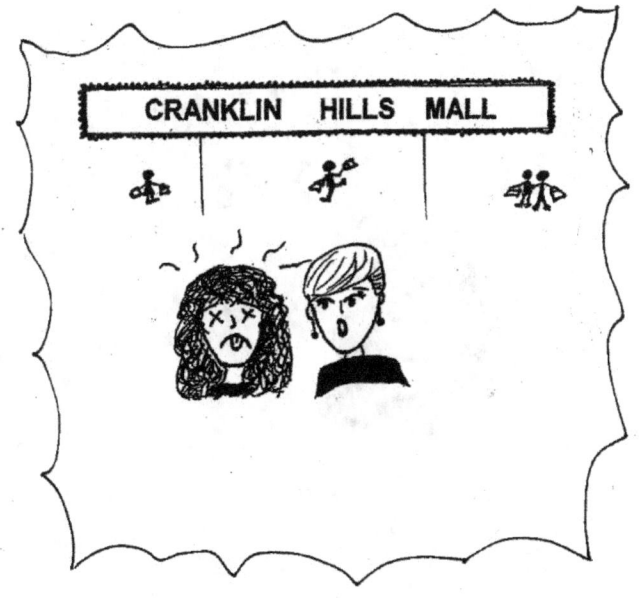

My friend was late,
so I bought a home
pregnancy test.

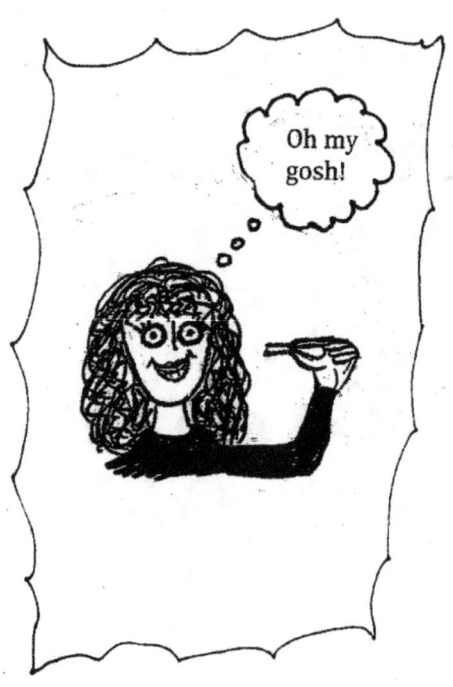

I had to be sure, so I
went to my doctor to
have a blood test.

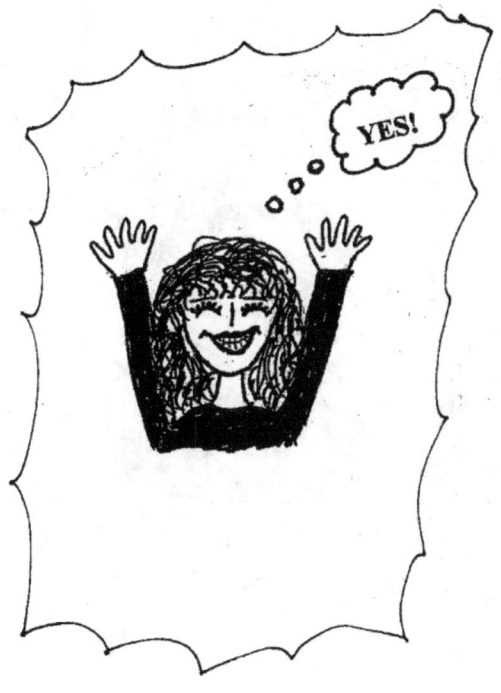

I told my guy on a
special evening.
He was so happy!

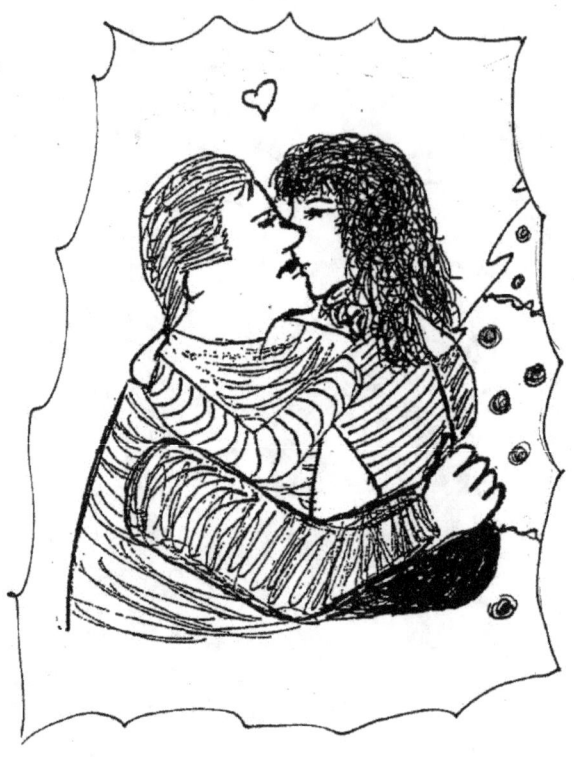

My family was thrilled!

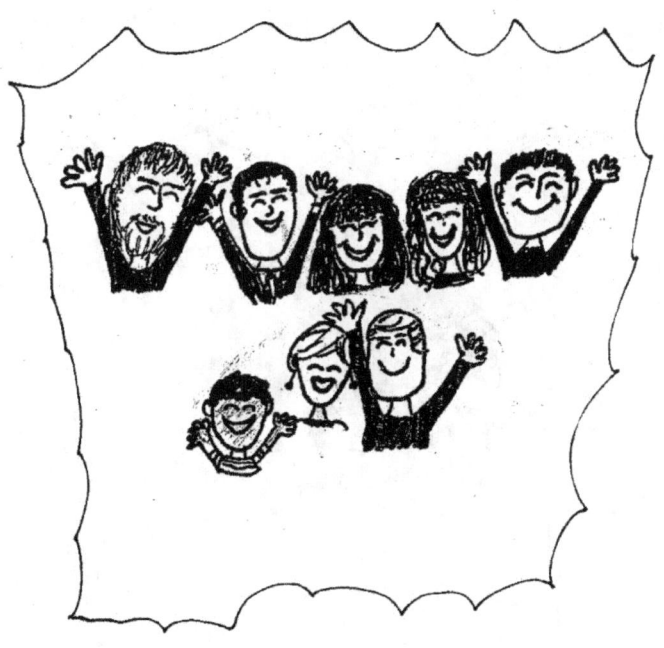

And so was I!

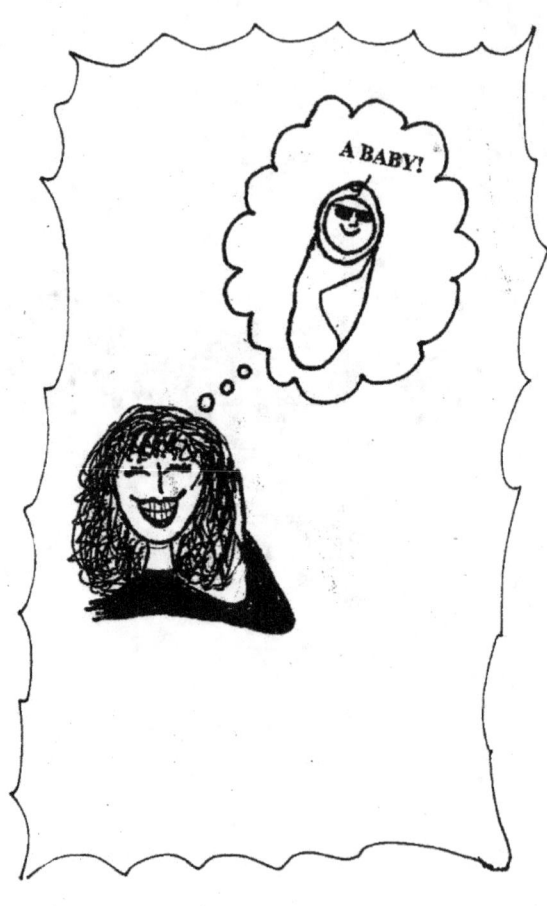

Then, came the morning
sickness.

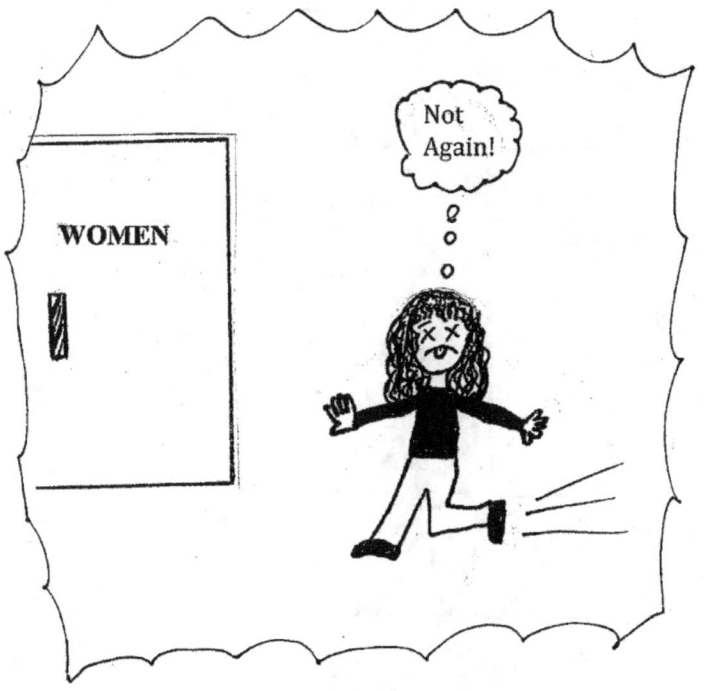

One thing that kept me
cool while I was pregnant
is that I didn't complain
a lot.  Believe me, there
was plenty to complain
about, but I kept thinking
of the end result, a
beautiful baby!

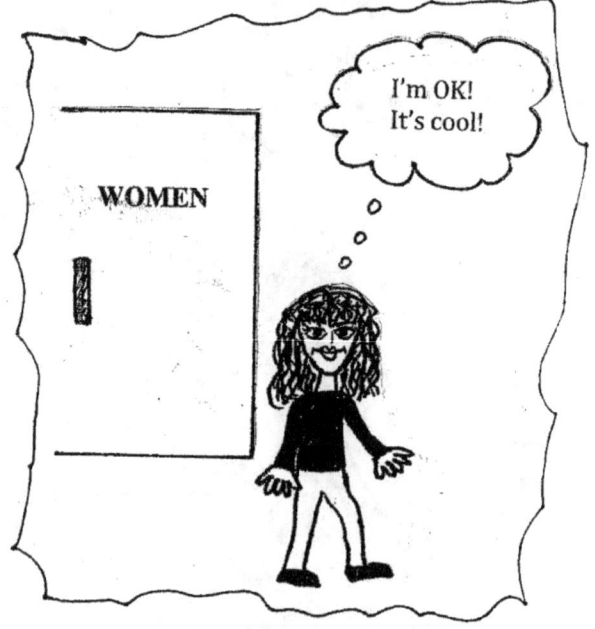

COOL TIP #1...
DON'T COMPLAIN
TOO MUCH.

When you are pregnant
you will go through
trimesters. The first
three months of
pregnancy are called the
first trimester. During
this time I was very
tired.

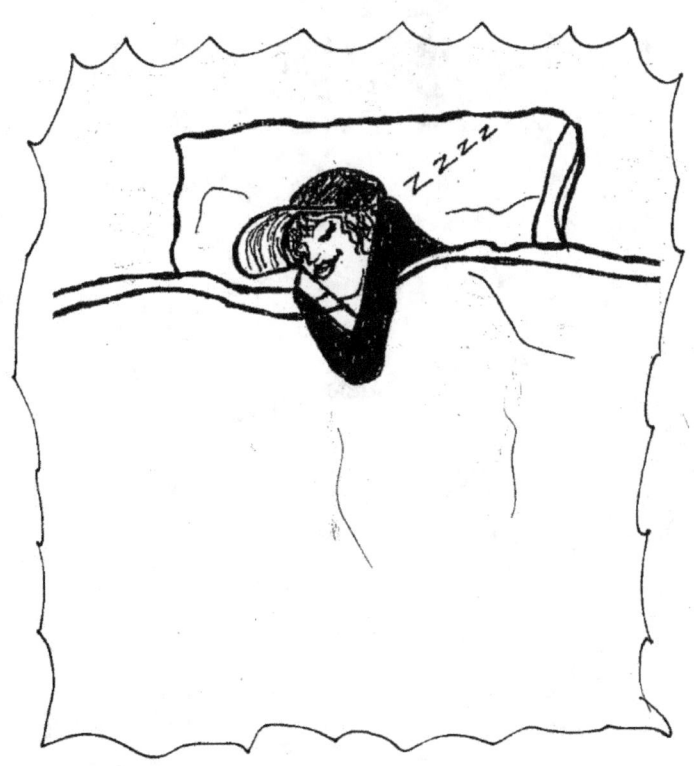

The first trimester can
be very overwhelming.
There were many things
that I loved and had to
stop...cold turkey!

NO SMOKING  NO DIET SODA

NO ALCOHOL  NO COFFEE

NO LIFTING HEAVY WEIGHTS

NO WATERCRAFT RIDING

NO AMUSEMENT RIDES

NO TANNING BEDS

# But I didn't complain too much.

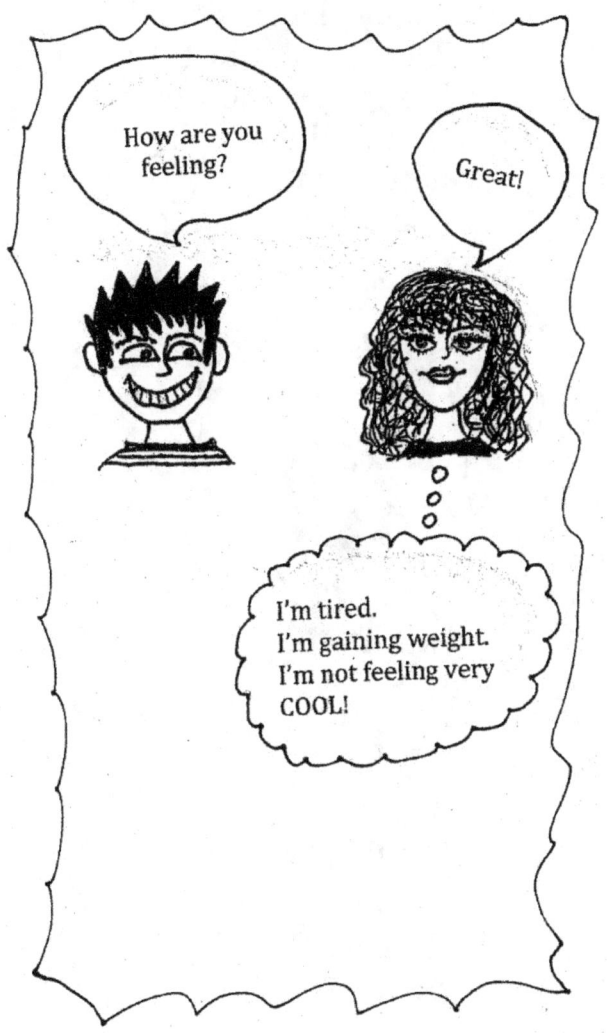

Months four, five and six
are called the second
trimester. During this
time I felt great but, I
started to gain some weight.
Finding cool maternity
clothes can be a
challenge.

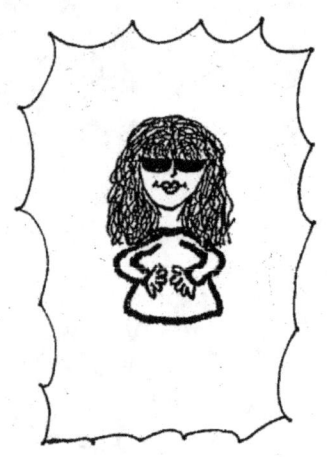

COOL TIP #2...
BUY COOL
MATERNITY
CLOTHES.

Look for XXX large or one
size fits all tee shirts.

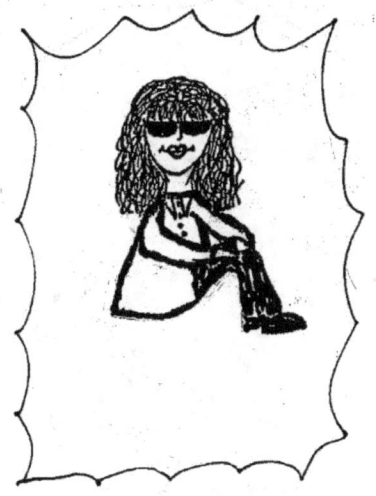

My guys' shirts made
cool maternity tops.

# Here are some other cool maternity clothes.

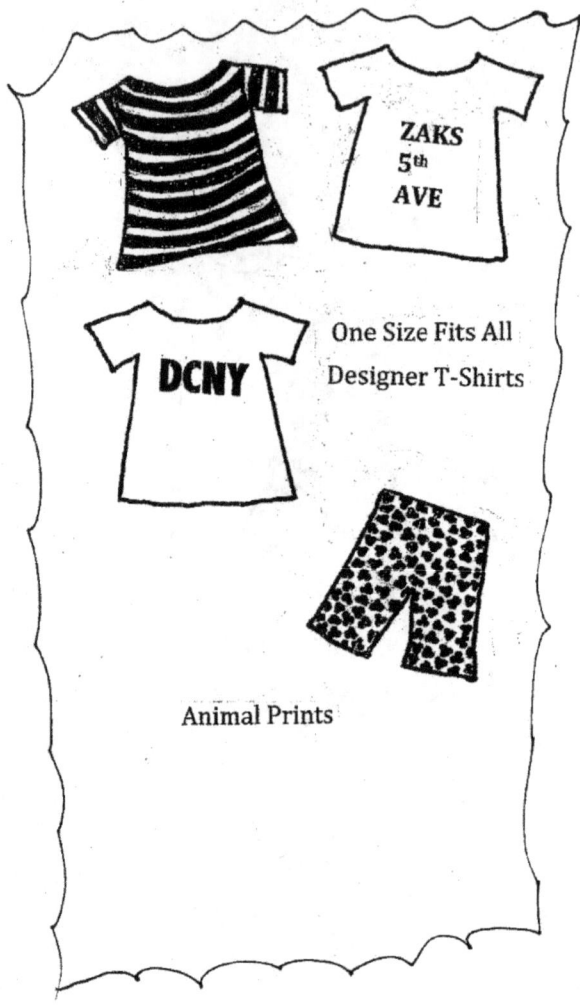

ZAKS
5th
AVE

One Size Fits All
Designer T-Shirts

DCNY

Animal Prints

Warmer maternity clothes...
try leggings and a big
sweater.  Very cool.

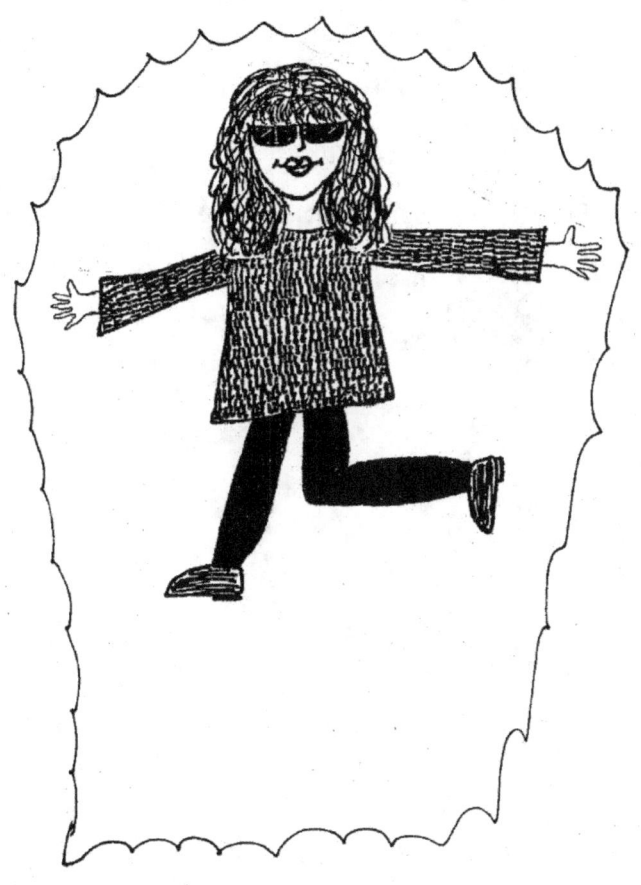

# Also, accessorize like crazy!

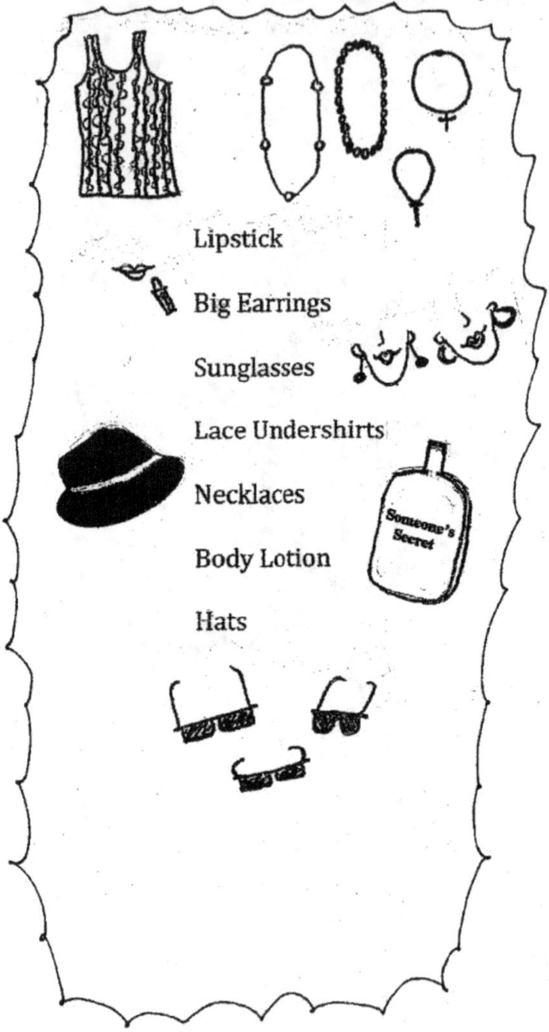

Lipstick

Big Earrings

Sunglasses

Lace Undershirts

Necklaces

Body Lotion

Hats

When you are pregnant, you
will have an ultrasound. This
allows you to see the baby,
without the hazards of an x-ray.
It also helps the doctor verify
the due date and make sure
everything is growing normally.

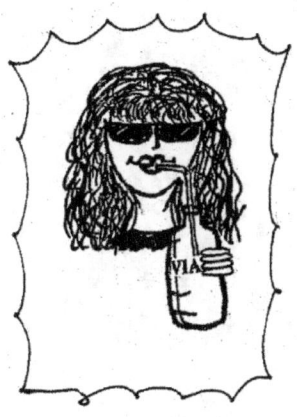

First, you drink a lot of water.
A full bladder is necessary for
the abdominal exam.

Then, you wait in the doctor's office and pray he's not running late.

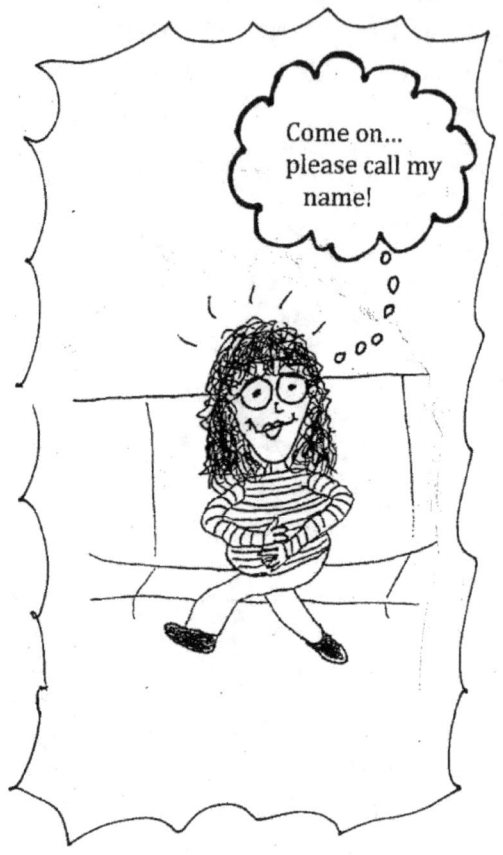

When your bladder is nice
and full, the technician
presses on your stomach,
to take measurements and
pictures of the baby.

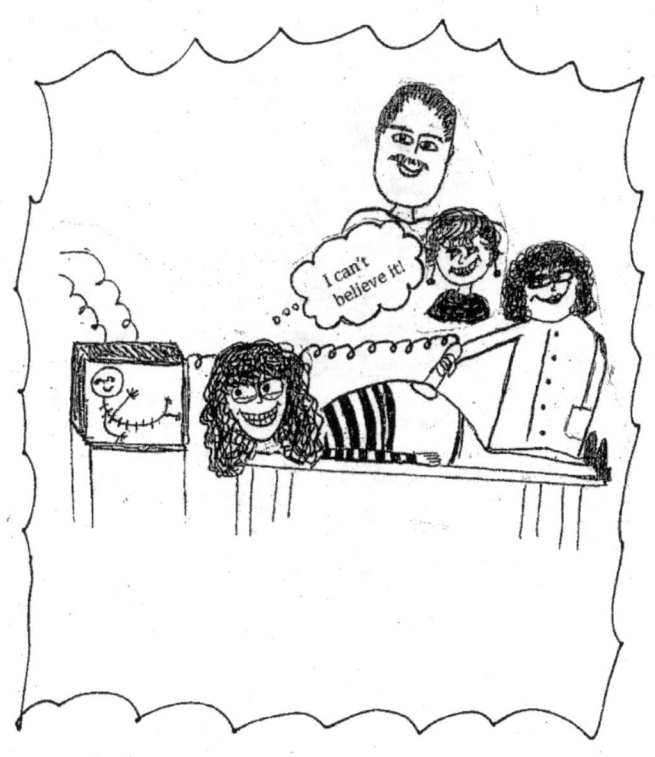

After the pictures are
taken, you RUN to the
restroom.

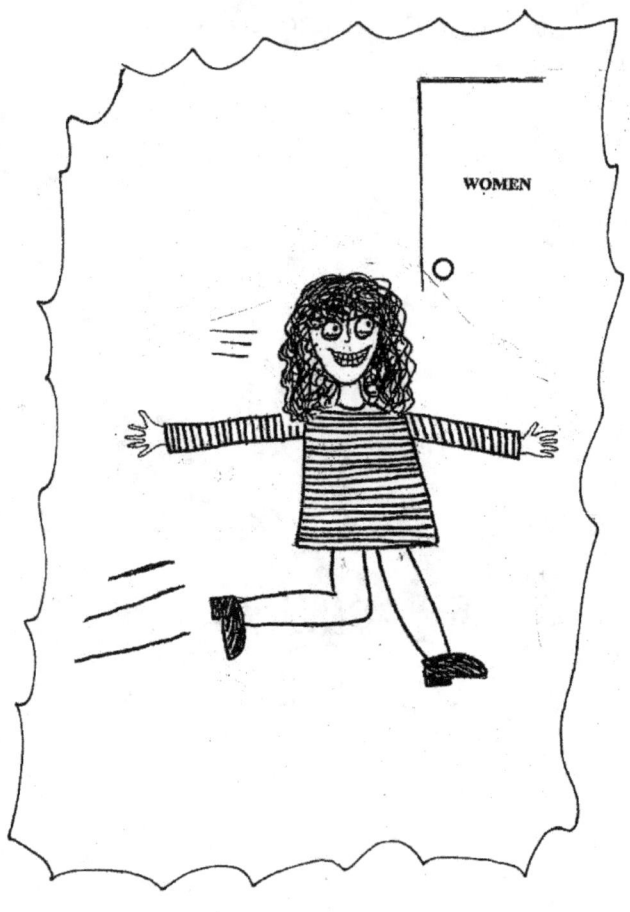

# COOL TIP #3...
# EXERCISE AND
# EAT RIGHT.

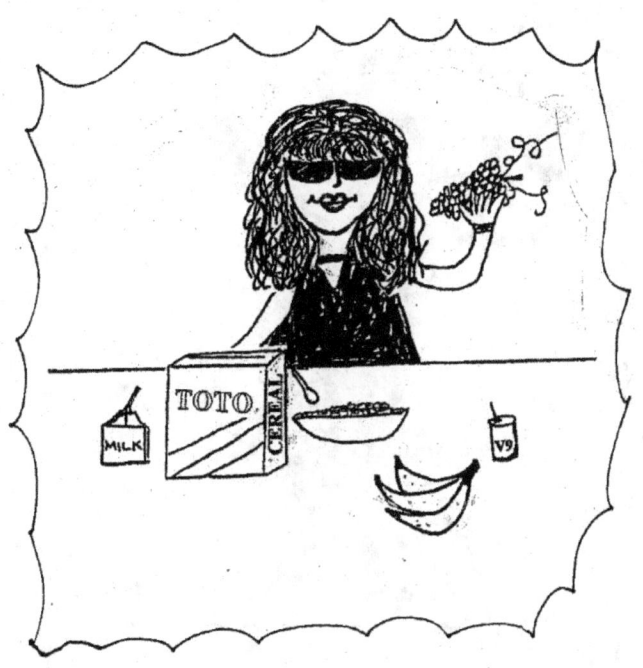

I was determined to
keep fit while I was
pregnant.  I ate a well
balanced diet and
walked on the treadmill,
five days a week.

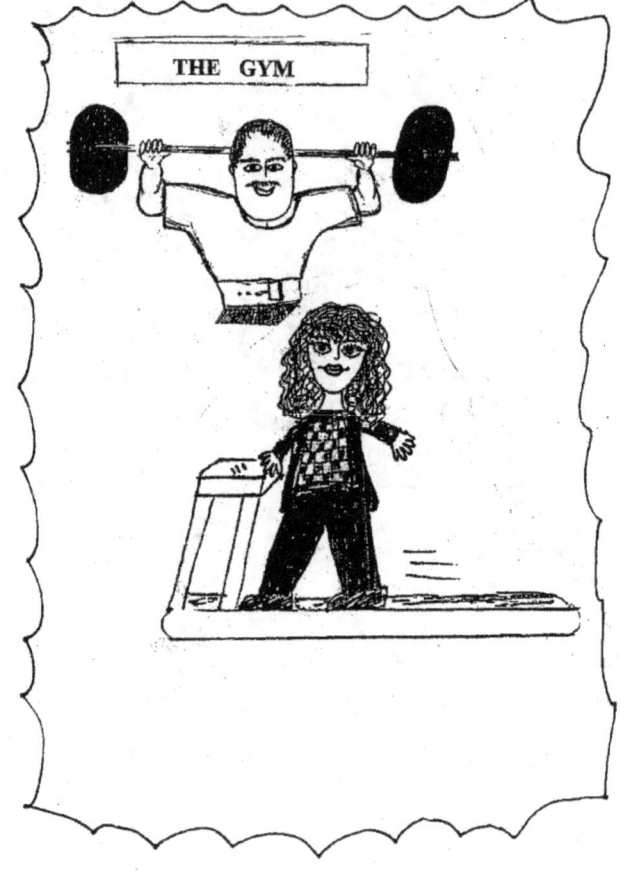

While you are pregnant, you may have a hard time keeping your hair looking cool.  Sure, your hair grows in thicker because of the vitamins you're taking but, what about the color?  NO hair dyes, bleaching or chemicals.  There's only one solution...get a cool haircut!

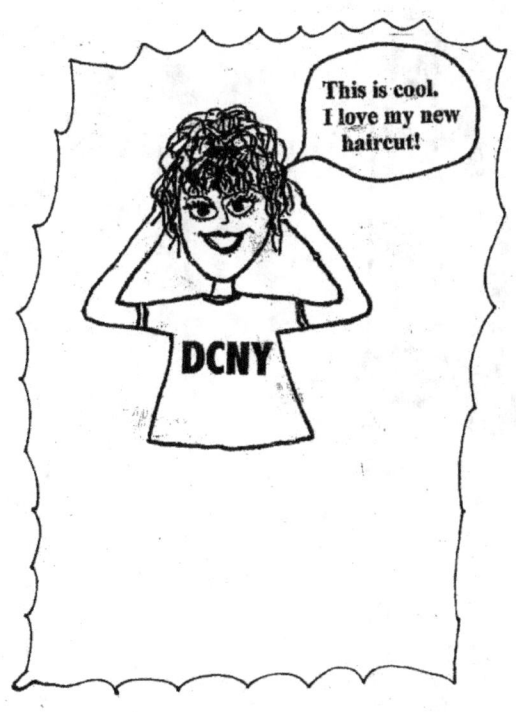

Each month, my body
changed a little more.

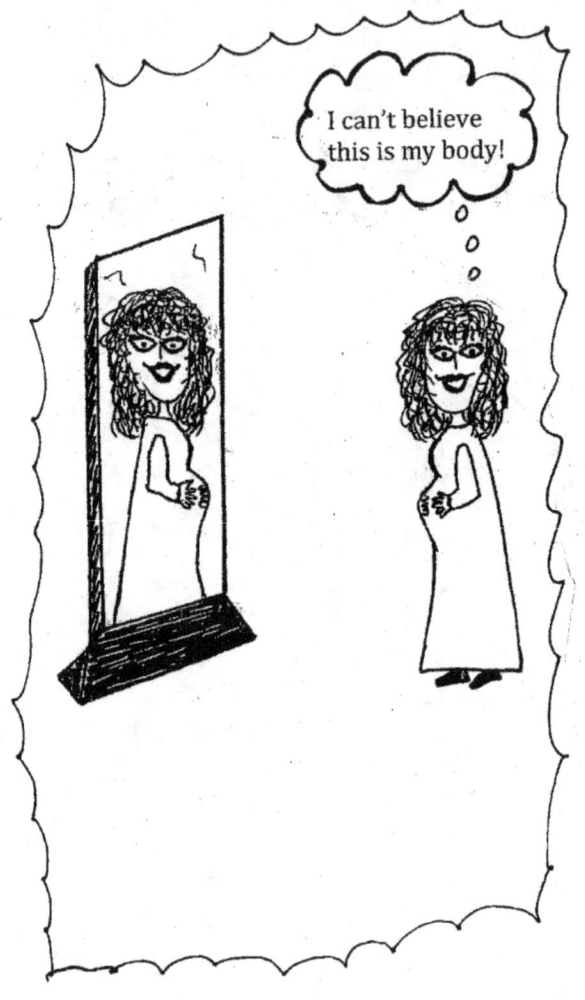

Not only did I have to deal
with my stomach getting bigger,
I had a dark line appear down
the middle of it!  Dark spots
appeared on my face.  This
was all caused by pregnancy
hormones.  I have two words
to say about that...cover-up!
Don't worry...they will fade
after delivery!

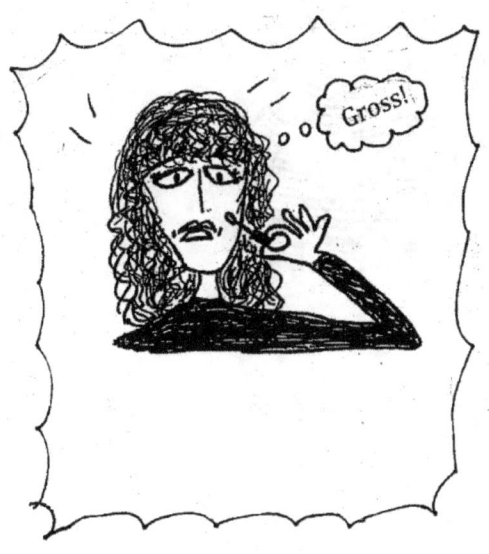

No one ever told me that
my belly button was going
to pop out.

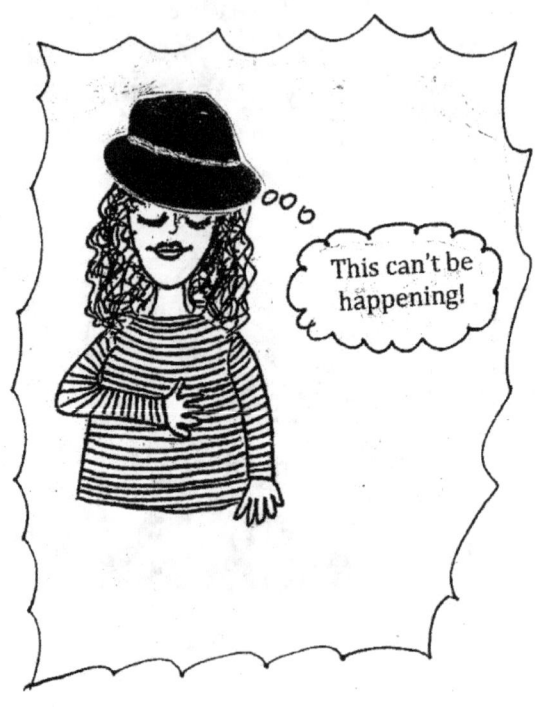

COOL TIP #4...
USE A SMALL PIECE OF
WATERPROOF TAPE ON
YOUR BELLY BUTTON.

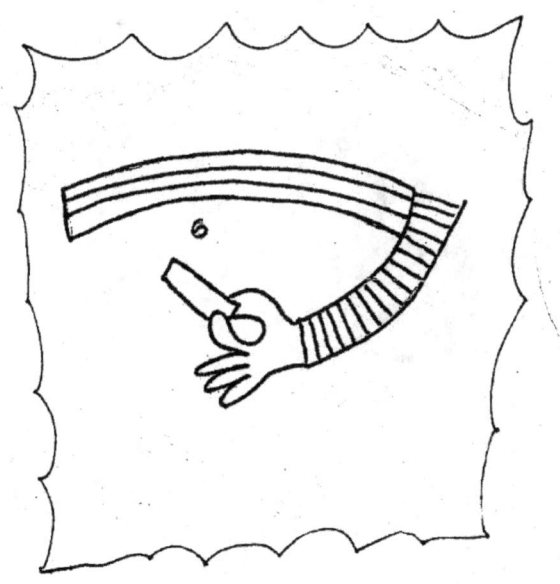

Months seven, eight and
nine are the third and
last trimester. This is
when you really grow!

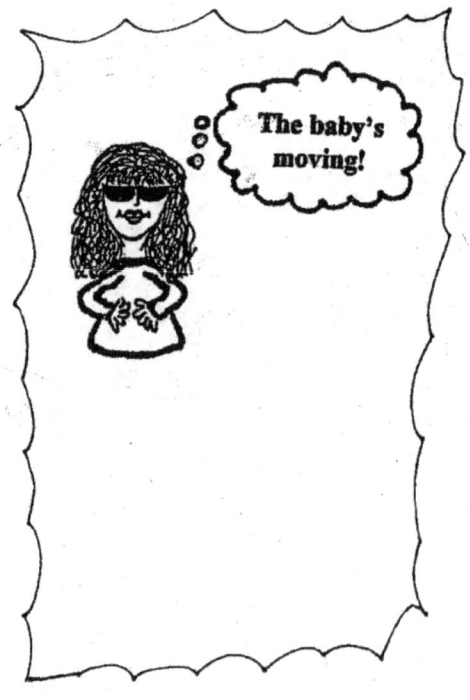

As your body expands, stick with buying bigger bikini underwear. How could you possibly feel cool wearing this?

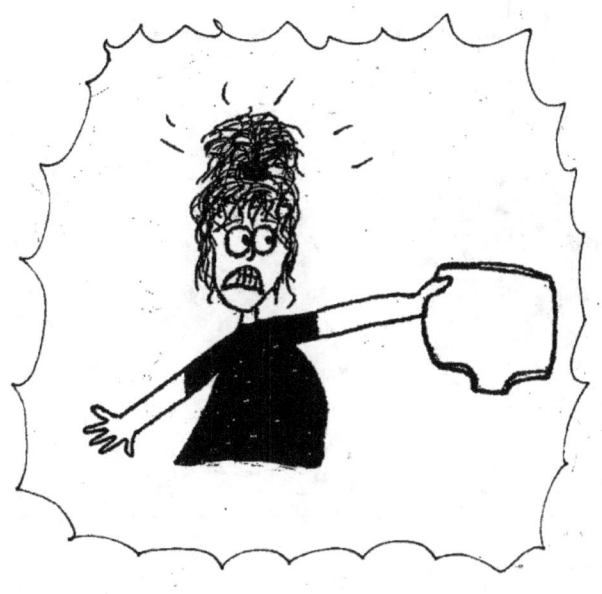

As my stomach grew,
some people could not
keep their hands off of it!

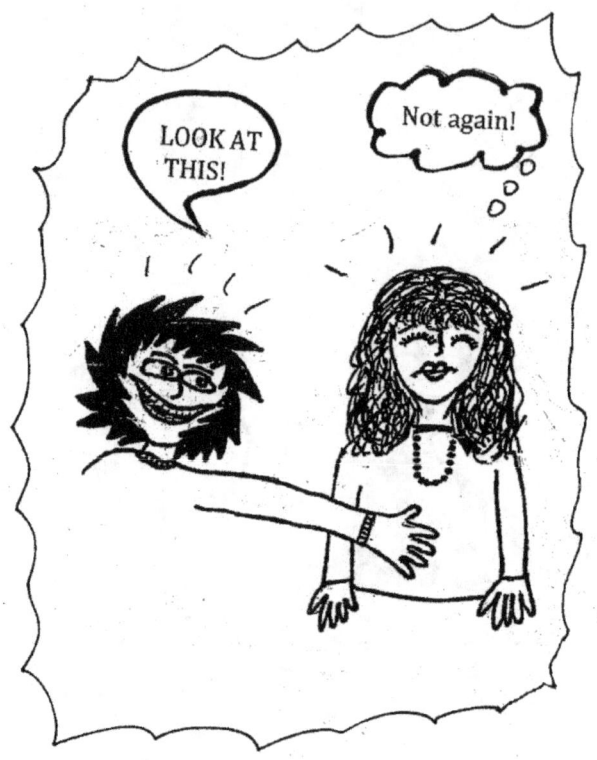

And everyone had
a story.

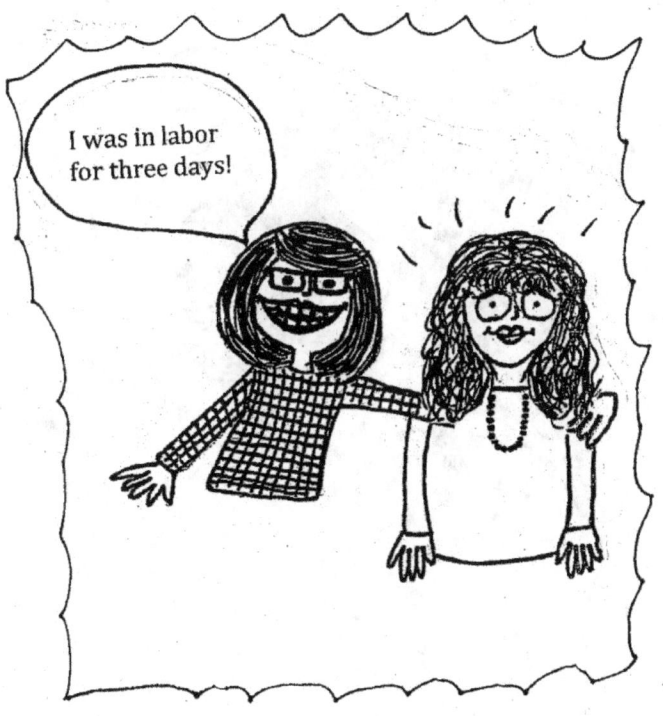

And everyone had
a comment.

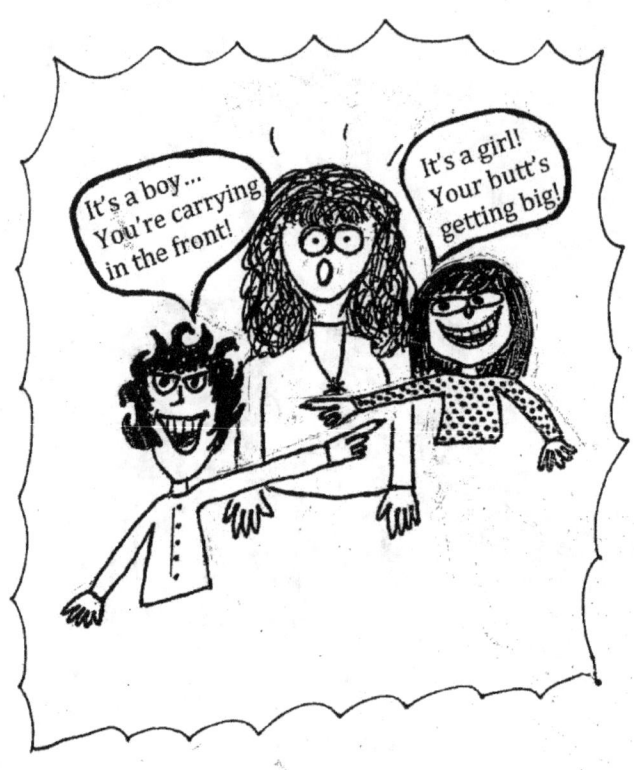

No matter what stories
you hear, remember
COOL TIP #5...
KEEP YOUR
SENSE OF HUMOR!

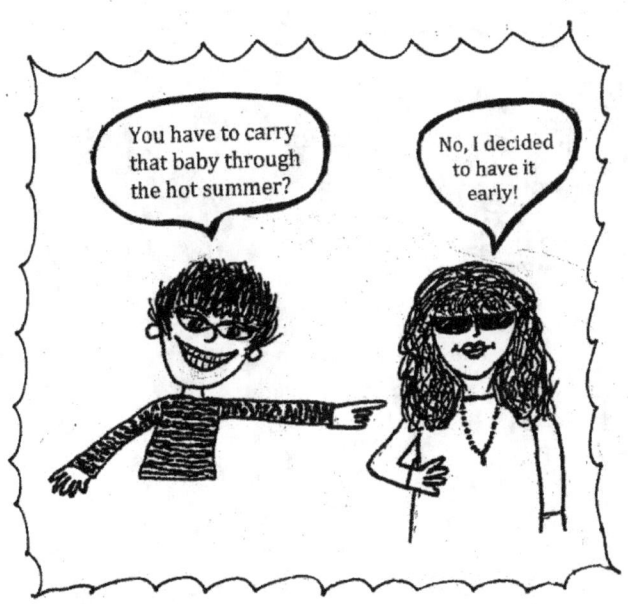

My guy and I attended childcare classes together. These classes helped us a lot!

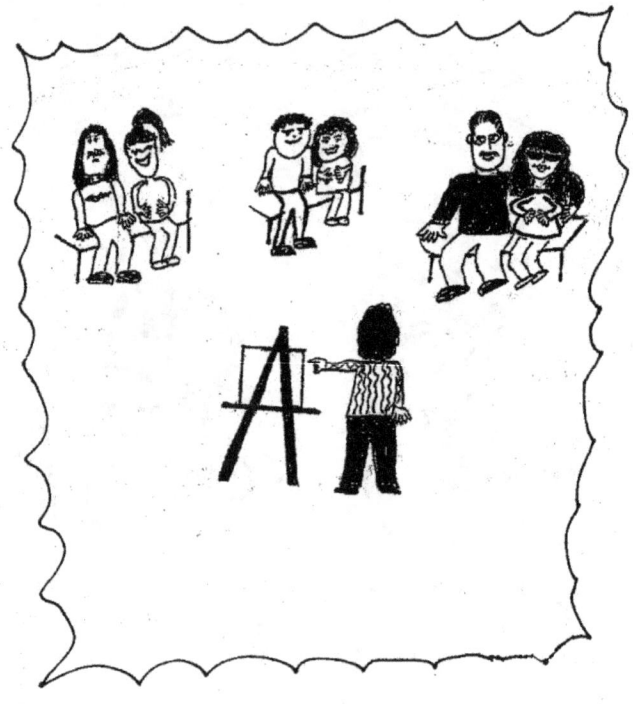

We also read books
and magazines.

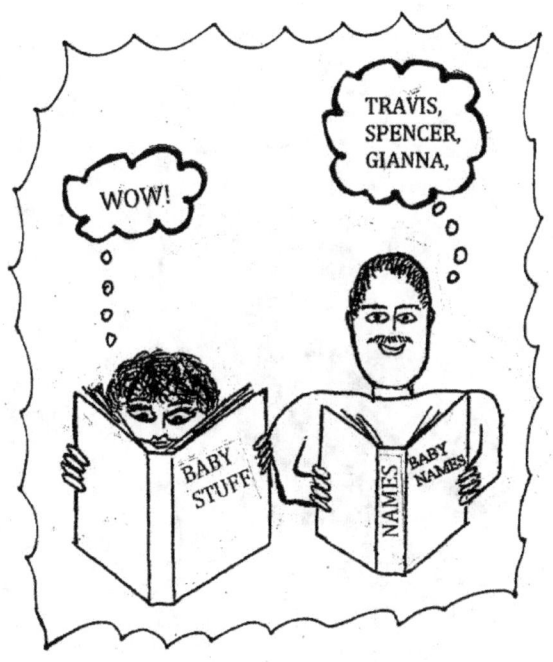

I never knew what
heartburn felt like
until I was
pregnant!  Yuck!

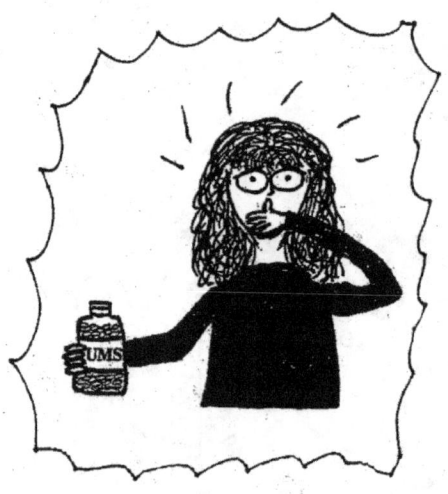

Sometimes my back
would ache really badly!
COOL TIP #6...
A COOL GEL PACK
HELPS SOOTHE
BACK PAIN.
You could also get your
guy to massage your back.

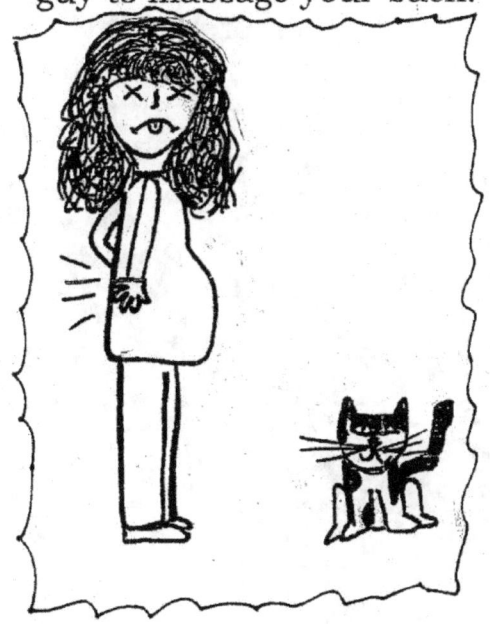

# COOL TIP #7...
# HAVE YOUR
# OVERNIGHT
# BAG PACKED.

You just never know when you will be going to the hospital  Don't forget a hat.  Your hair can look pretty silly after laying in a hospital bed for a few hours!

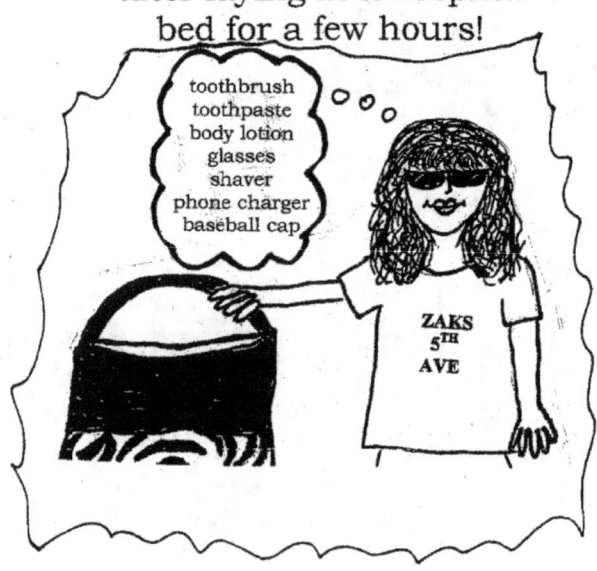

COOL TIP #8...
KEEP SMILING.
I learned this tip
from my mom.
If you look happy,
people seem to be
nicer to you.

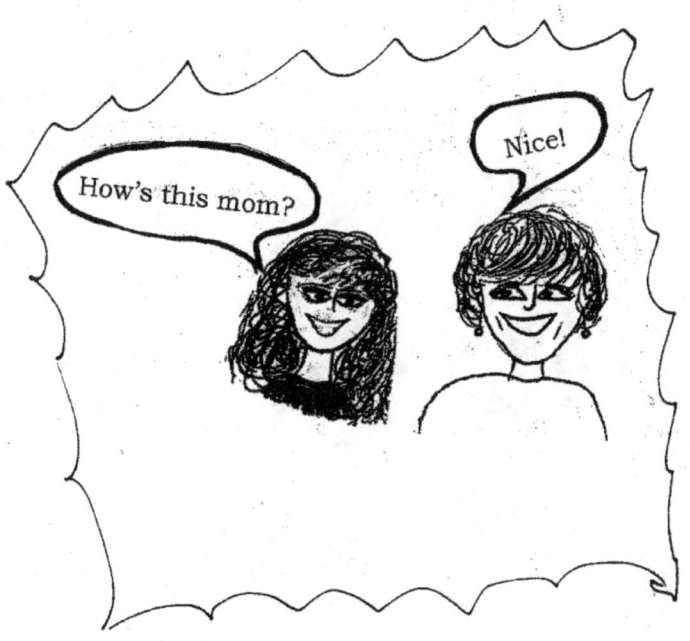

COOL TIP #9...
KEEP YOURSELF
LOOKING GOOD.
Do your hair and make-up
every day. And, don't forget
to keep your legs smooth,
even if you have to
do this lying down.

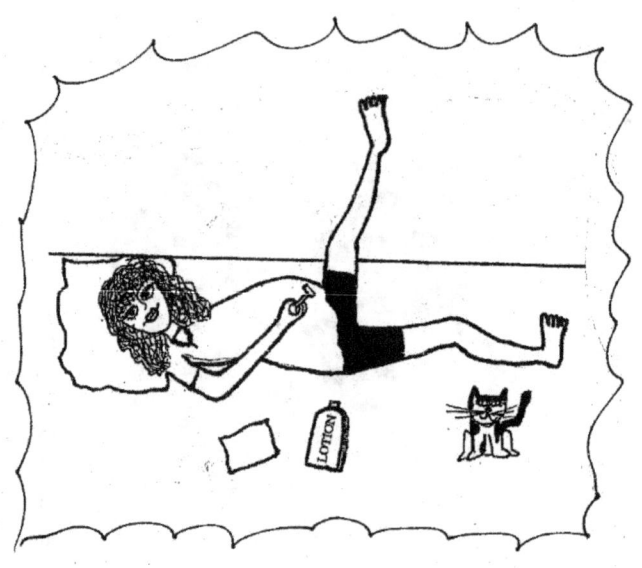

One morning during
my ninth month,
my water broke.

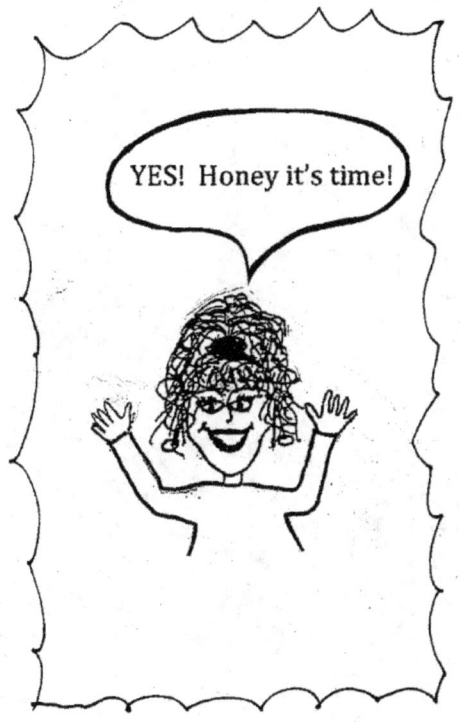

I called my doctor,
finished shaving my
legs and putting on
my make-up, and we
were off to the hospital.

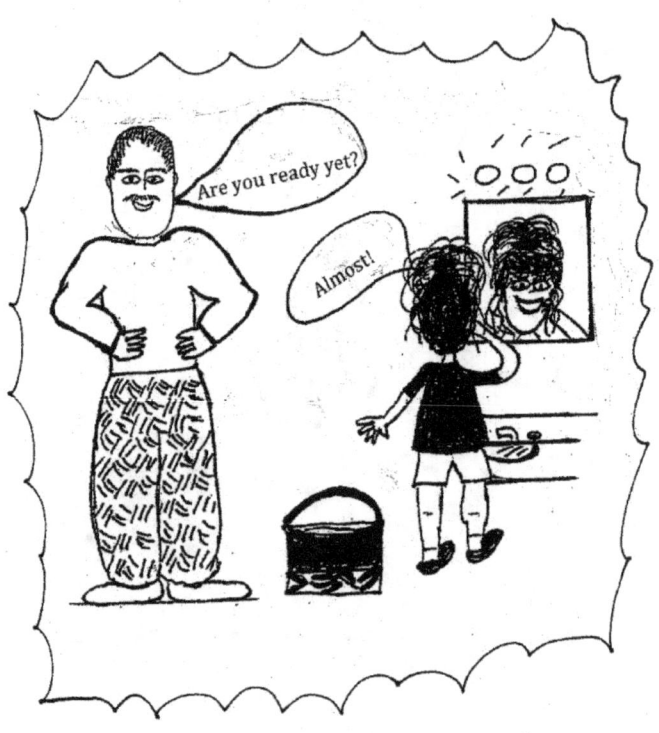

# COOL TIP #10...
## BRING COOL SOCKS IN CASE YOUR FEET GET COLD.

Hospital booties aren't that cool.

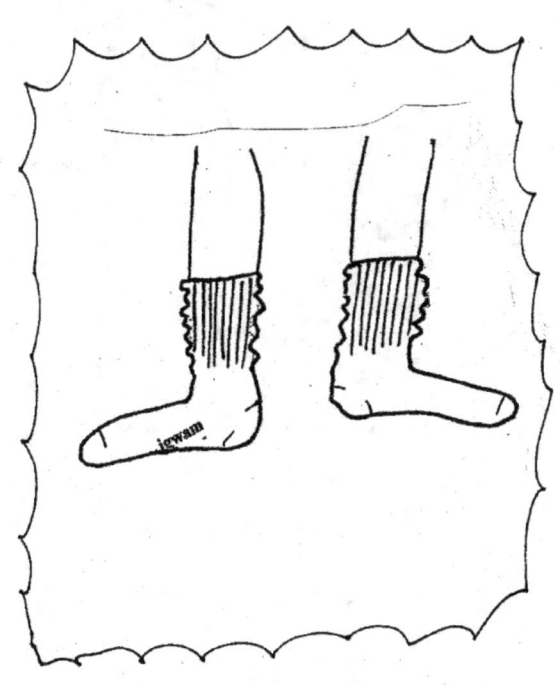

My guy was a
great coach!

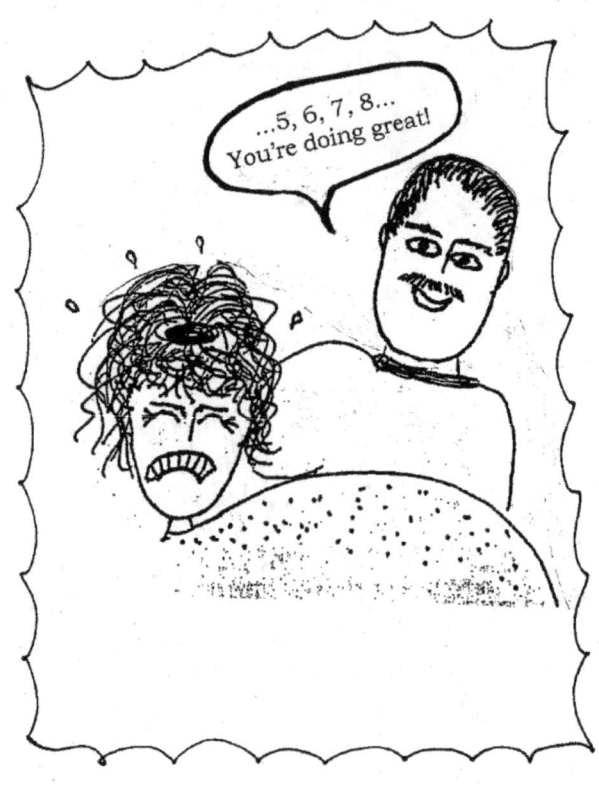

Just before the baby
was born, my mom
and sister were
allowed to come in.

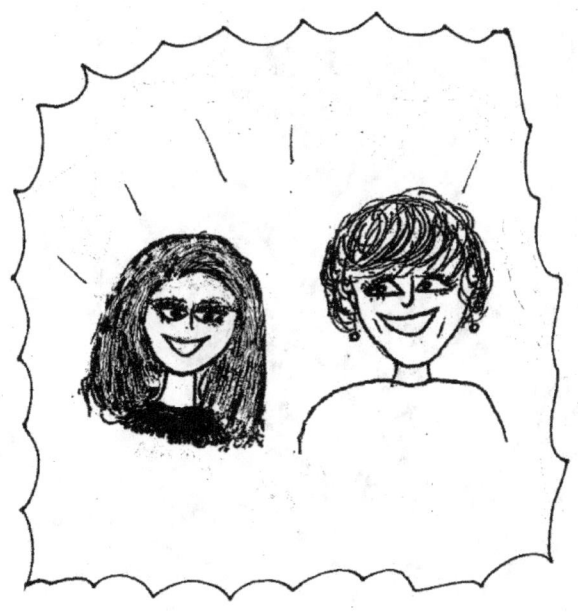

When my baby was born,
My doctor said,
"It's a boy!"

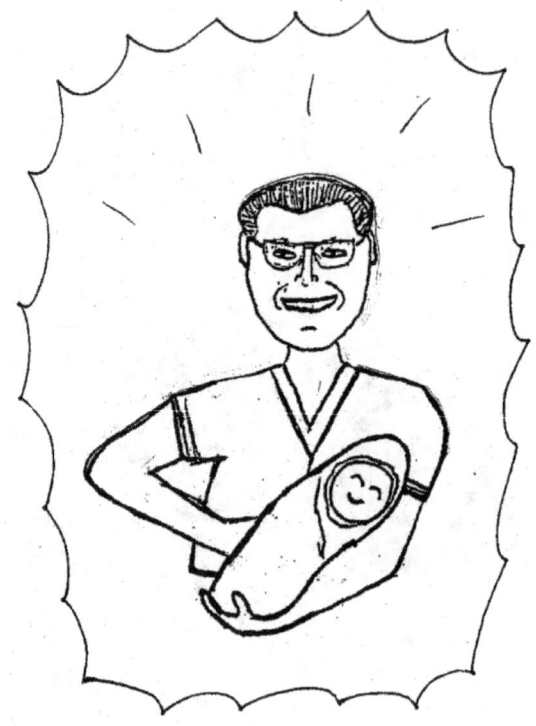

My baby was born on his
grandfather's birthday.

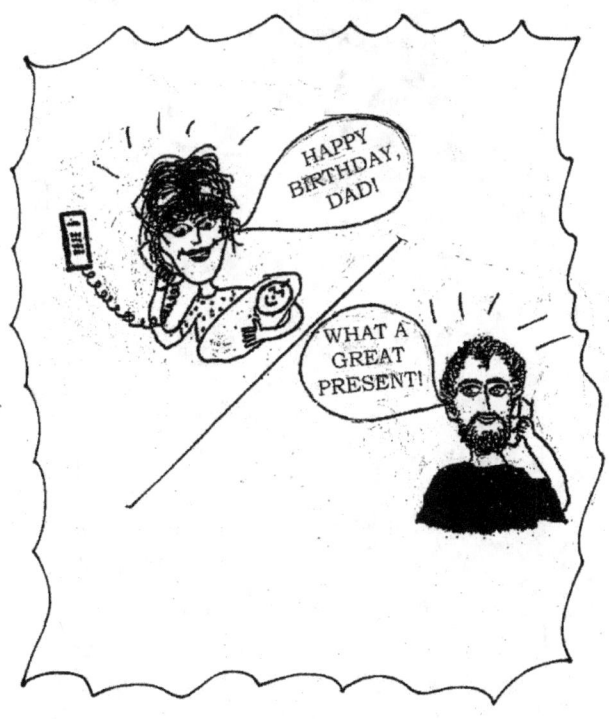

The End...

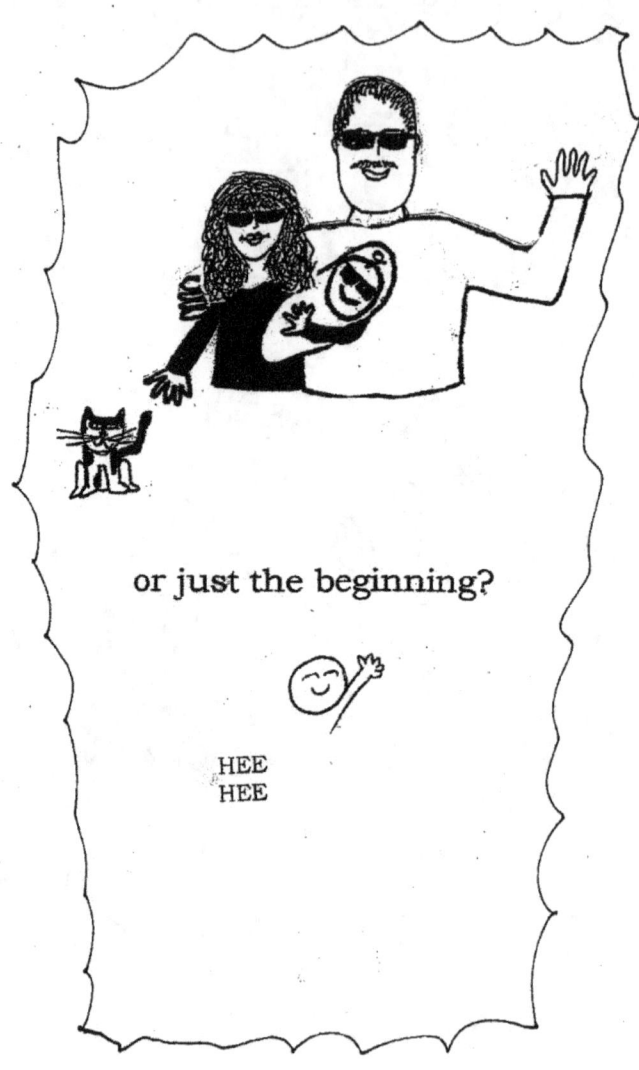

or just the beginning?

HEE
HEE

www.ingramcontent.com/pod-product-compliance
Lightning Source LLC
Chambersburg PA
CBHW060230290526
45789CB00003B/1491